Moving Beyond Depression:

A Step by Step System for Reclaiming Your Life From Depression

Carol L Rickard, LCSW

Well YOUniversity® Publications

Copyright © 2011 Carol L. Rickard

All rights reserved.

ISBN: 09821010-1-5
ISBN-13: 978-0-9821010-1-8

Moving Beyond Depression
by Carol L Rickard, LCSW

© Copyright 2008 Well YOUniversity Publications

ISBN 13: 978-0-9821010-1-8

All rights reserved. No part of this book may be reproduced for resale, redistribution, or any other purposes (including but not limited to eBooks, pamphlets, articles, video or audiotapes, & handouts or slides for lectures or workshops). Permission to reproduce these materials for those and any other purposes must be obtained in writing from the author.

The author & publisher of this book do not dispense medical advice nor prescribe the use of this material as a form of treatment. The author & publisher are not engaged in rendering psychological, medical, or other professional services.

The purpose of this material is educational only. Please see you doctor concerning any medical advice you may need.

Well YOUniversity, LLC

5 Zion Road, Hopewell, NJ 08525

www.WellYOUniversity.com

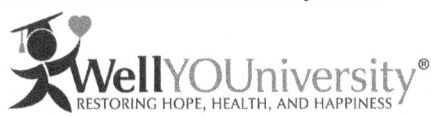

What you will get out of this book?!

- ✓ A proven system for creating healthy changes in your life.

- ✓ Being better able to **manage depression** rather than *it* manage you!

- ✓ A way of tracking and measuring your wellness foundation.

- ✓ Improved quality of life!

Contents

Introduction

What Makes It Different?	1
About This Book	2
My Own Story	4

The Wellness Blueprint: My Secret Weapon!

Chapter 1	What It Is! What It Is Not!	9
Chapter 2	Taking A Look At The Blueprint	11

Building the Foundation Corners!

Chapter 3	Medication	26
Chapter 4	Outpatient Follow-up	30
Chapter 5	Sobriety	35
Chapter 6	Structure	37

Building the Rest of the Foundation!

Chapter 7	Nutrition	41
Chapter 8	Exercise	45
Chapter 9	Support	48
Chapter 10	Socialization	52
Chapter 11	Coping Skills	56
Chapter 12	Communication	60
Chapter 13	Spirituality	64
Chapter 14	Leisure	68
Chapter 15	Acceptance	71
Chapter 16	Self Esteem	75
Chapter 17	Putting It All Together!	80

Bonus	82
Additional Resources	83
About Well YOUniversity, LLC	85

What Makes It Different?

This book is like none you may have seen!

It is specifically designed for the person who is experiencing **depression**

One of the most frustrating symptoms is **poor concentration & memory**.

This makes it very hard for people to *READ*...

But not this book!

Two things make this book different:

1) There is limited amount of text on each page.

2) I use a lot of pictures. Brains remember pictures! (Especially when depressed)

About This Author

Over the past 17 years I have had the opportunity to help **1,000's** of people reclaim their lives from depression.

It has always been my belief that those who ended up being hospitalized were the lucky ones!

It gave them the opportunity to learn about depression & develop the **tools needed to manage it.**

This gave them a tremendous advantage over people who were in outpatient treatment and not offered those same learning opportunities.

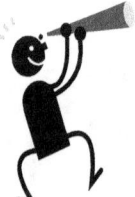 It has always been my **dream** to one day teach the rest of the world those tools!

I created **Well YOUniversity** to do just that!

This book is designed to give you the "tools" to reclaim your life from depression.

How do I know these tools work?

I have had to **live what I teach** in order to reclaim my own life from depression that once threatened to "*bury me alive*"

I believe the plan I developed & am about to share with you is what has helped me

get well & stay well!

What makes my work different is that I tend to teach with pictures as well as words.

I think an episode of depression is like an avalanche – We get **buried** underneath it. Just as with an avalanche, most times we need help digging out!

My goal with this book is to give you **the "shovel"** to start doing that!

My Own Story

My battle with depression started as a teenager, although I wouldn't come to realize that until many years later….

During the early 1990's, I had been going to see my primary care doctor every 3-4 months

&

kept getting tested for mono.

I was always so tired and had no energy.

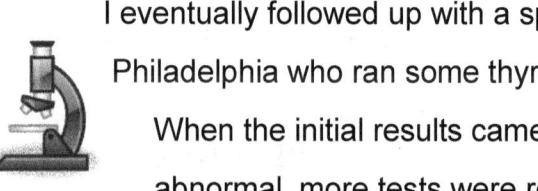

I eventually followed up with a specialist in Philadelphia who ran some thyroid tests. When the initial results came back abnormal, more tests were required.

Those came back showing there was **nothing wrong.** I was relieved & upset at the same time.

I remembering thinking,

'What is wrong with me?'

Then one day I was sitting in doctor's rounds at the psychiatric hospital where I' started working 9 months earlier as a recreation therapist.

I learned something that
changed my life forever!

The doctor was explaining how an abnormal **TSH** test could be a possible indicator of depression.

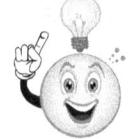

'That was it!' I thought to myself.

Later that day I called my internist & made an appointment. It was the beginning of my recovery!

She agreed with my idea it was **depression** I was experiencing & referred me to a psychiatrist.

From my work, I had come to learn medication was going to be important part of getting well.

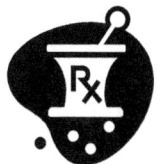

During the early time of trying to get a medication to

stabilize my mood, I found myself sinking further in to

the black hole.

Most days,
    I could pull my self together to function
well enough to get through my work hours, but it
would take all I had just to drive home & climb in to bed.

I was so exhausted….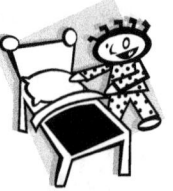

Some days, I couldn't do it.
I would get to work & have to leave.

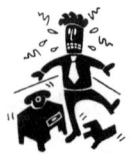 I couldn't hold myself together enough
to be professional around my patients.

Thank goodness I had a supportive director.

During that same time, I remember several times
when I found myself ***having thoughts about death***.

I wasn't feeling suicidal. It was more the thoughts of

something happening to cause my own death, however not by my doing.

The one that stands out most in my mind was the time I had gone to the symphony on a date.

While I was sitting there, I found my self thinking:

'What if a gunman was to suddenly open fire on the audience? Could I hide myself in the bathroom & be safe?'

After a moment or two, I was able to pull my attention back to reality.

I knew then the depression really had me and it was going to take a fight to get my life back!

But I knew **recovery was possible!**

I had seen it happen…..MANY TIMES!!

So I started focusing on and identifying the factors in the hospital I believed helped people get well.

I also focused on the factors that seemed to lead to *relapse and people's re-hospitalization.*

From there……..

I developed my recovery plan
&
started living by it!

It is the same system I live by today!

Over the years I have shared this system with many.

Today I share it with you!

The Wellness Blueprint: My Secret Weapon!

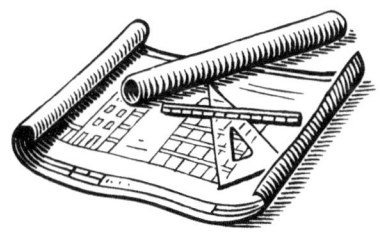

#1) What It Is! What It Is Not!

What It Is!

The Wellness Blueprint™ is a structured system that helps people rebuild & reclaim their lives from depression.

As you will see, we **need** to do more than just take medications…….

Medication is *ONLY* 1 tool! There are many more!

My belief is this:

We are **NOT** responsible for our illness,
We *ARE* responsible for our RECOVERY!

Just as with any type of blueprint-

When we follow it ….. we end up with the same results every time!

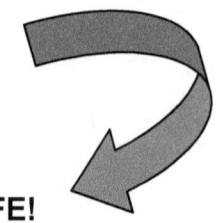

In this case — It's **QUALITY OF LIFE!**

What It Is Not!

The Blueprint is *not* a replacement for treatment with a professional healthcare provider.

Anybody using this book also needs to be connected to some type of healthcare professional for treatment of their mental health needs.

After all, the next important thing to having a blueprint to follow --

a responsible building CONTRACTOR to supervise the work!!

Even if you feel your mental health symptoms are mild, please talk to a healthcare provider about them.

IMPORTANT: If you or somebody you know is experiencing significant depression, have thoughts of death & dying or hurting themselves / others -

please contact your local crisis center or emergency room for immediate help.

#2)   Taking A Look at the Blueprint

I need you to imagine…

I am standing on this 4-legged chair right in front of you!

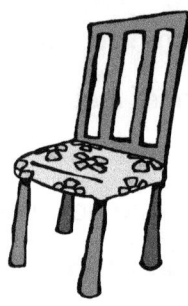

You saw off one of the legs….

What do you think will happen?   Do I fall on you?!

Probably not –

since I have 3 legs I can still shift my weight to!

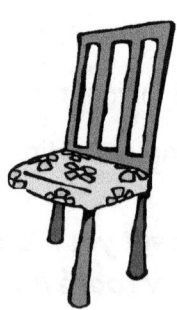

You saw off another one!

What happens now?!

Have you ever heard of STILTS?

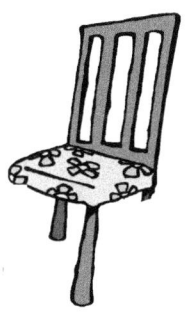

The truth is ....

I could only stay up on those things for a short time!

Even if I was good at stilts -
it wouldn't take much of a bump to knock me over.

(We all know **LIFE IS FULL OF BUMPS!**).

Now, you saw off the 3rd leg –

leaving me with only 1!!!!

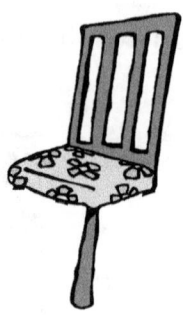

Guess what?   I'm going down…

Oops!

I never could pogo stick!

The key point here is:

When we rely just on medication to make us better…..

It is like trying to stay up on just 1 leg!

It doesn't work so well

Does it make sense to you that at the very least,

we *could* get away with 3 legs?

Think 3-legged stool!

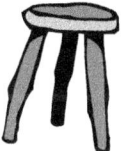

Now, if you have ever sat on a 3-legged stool

You are very aware they aren't too sturdy!!!

It's easy to loose your balance & tip over!

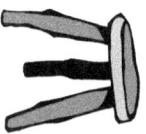

So,

We want to make sure that we have all 4 legs!

The Foundation Corners

Just as with any good structure,

wellness must be built on solid *foundation corners*.

The foundation corners of the Wellness Blueprint™ are!

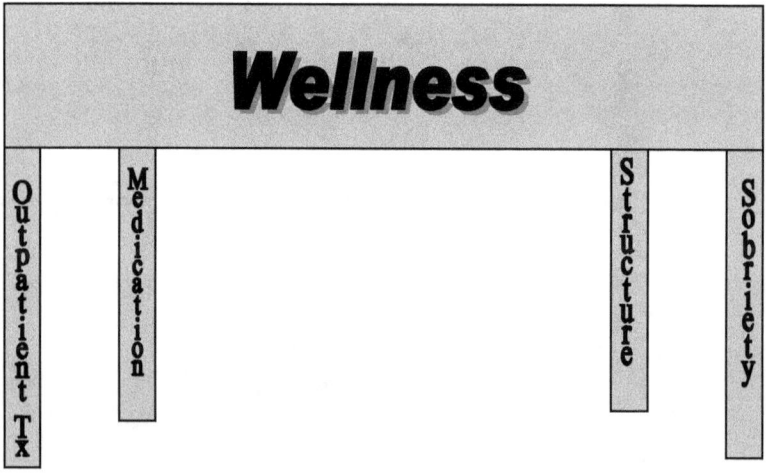

We'll go in to detail about each of these in a few pages!

Before we work on building the rest of the foundation…

We must concentrate on these corners.

It is important to make these a **priority!!**

This means there is no messing around

when it comes to these areas!!

Do not miss doses of your medicine…..

Do not miss appointments….

Do not mix alcohol or other drugs with medications….

Do not spend your day in bed….

The sooner you get these corners in place,

The sooner you will be on the way to building

your Wellness Blueprint™!

The Rest of The Foundation

Let me share with you the other 10 areas that make up the remainder of our Wellness Blueprint™:

Wellness

- Nutrition
- Exercise
- Support
- Socialization
- Coping Skills
- Communication
- Spirituality
- Leisure
- Acceptance
- Self Esteem

Putting these things in to place in our lives *requires* some work!

But the PAYOFF is GREAT!

Now,

Imagine me standing on a chair with **14** legs!!!

Don't you agree that would give me a

"**solid**, "**strong**", "**stable**", "**sturdy**" foundation?!!

(This is how my health has been since 1993)

I like to think & teach that stress is like an earthquake!

It can really shake up our lives!

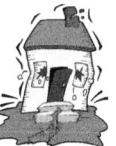

Foundations tend to take a bruising during earthquakes

and parts have been known to fall down.

We've got to make sure we have

enough of a foundation!

If we happen to lose some of it to

a big stressor going on in our lives....

We've got to have enough left to keep us **stable!**

The Domino Effect

Now,

it's important to understand how this foundation can

CRUMBLE!

under certain circumstances

&

lead to the depression returning again…

If you lose one of the four foundation corners……

it sets off a '*domino effect*' and the others start to fall.

It could be weeks, months, even years

before the depression starts to take over again…..

And believe me when it does return it

can be many times stronger than before.

There are **2** other ways to use the Wellness Blueprint™:

We use it to build a **ladder** so we can "**climb out of that big black hole**" we've been in….

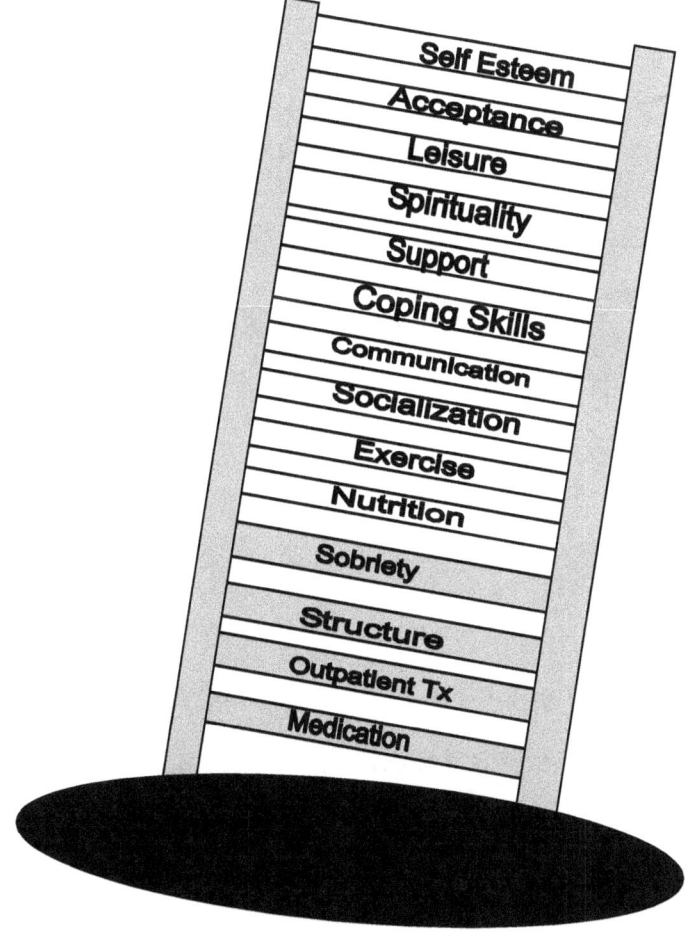

Or we use it to build a *cage* so we can keep that beast of an illness from running loose in our lives:

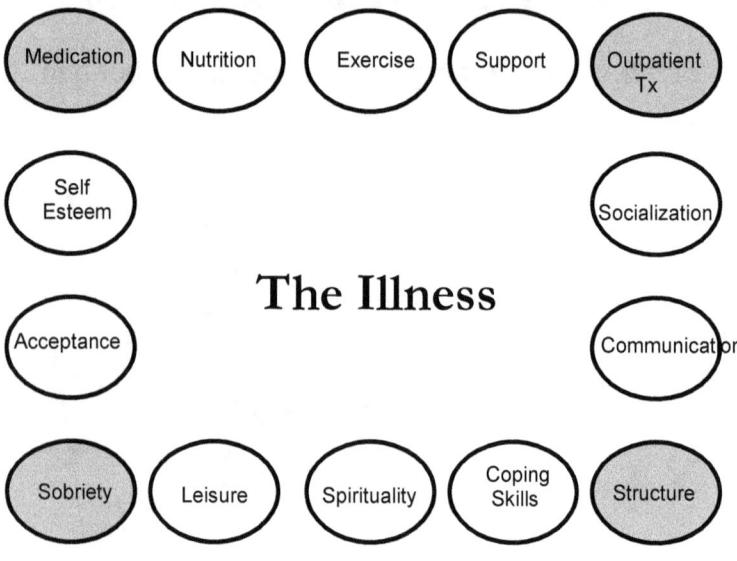

If medication is *not* a part of your life

please use the following amended blueprints!

No medications

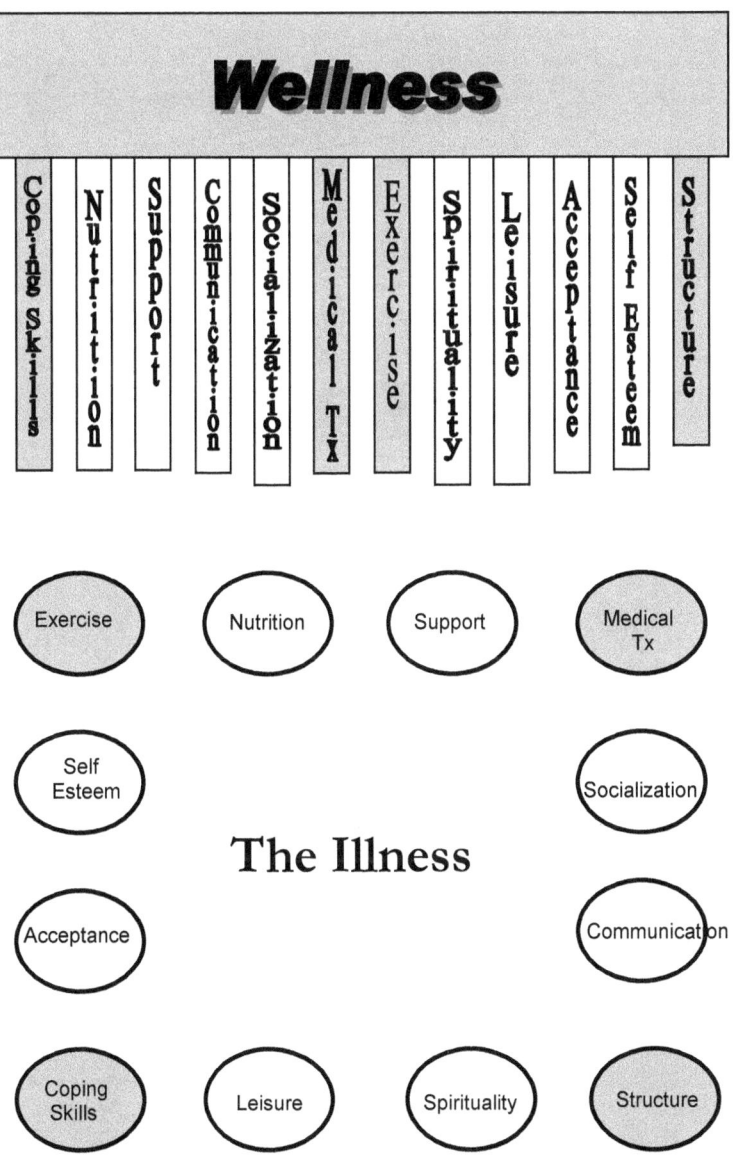

The ladder

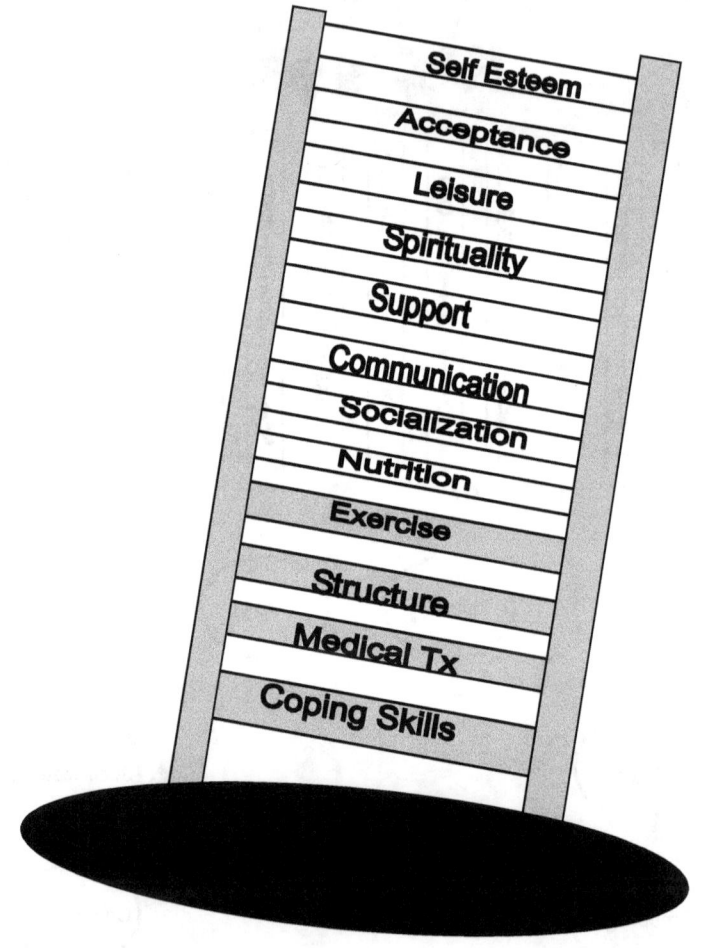

Building the Foundation Corners

#3) Medication

This can be one of the **hardest & most frustrating** part to get right.....

That's why it's IMPORTANT to have **many** of the other parts in place!

This is also a very personal area.

There are many people who don't believe in the use of psychiatric medications... or have family members who don't.

With respect to people's beliefs, I have *yet* to see someone whose symptoms have significantly impaired their ability to function in life get better without medication.

Therefore,

medication is an important part

of the Wellness Blueprint™.

We are fortunate to have so many **options**

these days when it comes to medications.

And although the **exact** scientific cause

of depression is yet to be determined,

advances in medicine & technology have offered

many more ways of

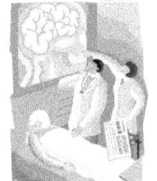

targeting symptoms & providing relief.

They are **far from perfect!**

&

worse yet,

don't work the same for everyone -

which makes it hard finding one that is helpful for you!

When it comes to taking **Medications** here are some things you can do that will make sure you stay depressed!!

Of course to get well you want to *do the opposite!*

To stay depressed:

✓ **MISS DOSES** & don't tell your prescriber.

✓ Run out of medication all together!

✓ Stop taking them!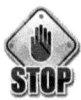

People can feel better & don't think they need them

or

still feel bad & don't think they are working!

✓ Drink alcohol -

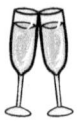 even a couple glasses of wine can be too much of a mix with medications.

✓ Start changing the amounts on your own!

Most important to getting well:

1. Don't let other people decide for you.

2. Take all medication as **prescribed!**

3. _Talk_ with your prescriber and _be honest._

4. Do not put M.D. after your name. Let the doctor make the changes!

A Personal Experience:

I remember the first medicine the psychiatrist put me on to treat my depression. I couldn't shut my mind off. I had butterflies in my stomach. I couldn't sleep until the very early hours of the morning… of course that was Saturday night! I remember taking the Sunday dose because I wouldn't stop it & put MD after my name! Fortunately, I was able to speak to her Monday & we tried another medication, which turned to be very helpful. (If I had to do it all over again – I'd call the doctor's service that same night I had that experience!)

#4) Outpatient Treatment

Resources for this vary from city to city, state to state, person to person. It all depends on where you live

&

what type of insurance you have, **if any**...

Can you imagine somebody with a broken bone not going to get follow-up treatment?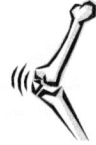

PROBABLY NOT LIKELY!

The same should hold true in dealing with our mental health.

Just because our **injury isn't visible** doesn't mean that it can go without treatment.

Outpatient treatment is best if you can see someone who is a mental health professional. It's important you have someone to talk with about problems and struggles in life.

This could be social workers, counselors, therapists, psychologists, & addiction counselors

We must also have **someone to prescribe medication**!

This includes psychiatrists & advanced practice nurses.

Because resources are often so limited – many people end up having their depression be managed by their **primary care doctor** or local clinic.

If you are in this type of situation

&

*feel your symptoms **are not** improving*

you might want to **ASK** for a referral to a psychiatrist.

Here's why: Suppose you had a Porsche & it needed some engine work

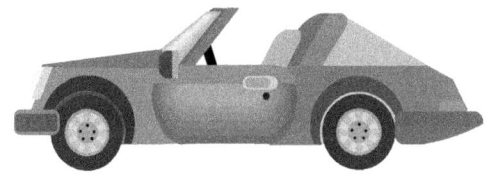

WHO WOULD YOU TAKE IT TO?

The Porsche Mechanic

or

The Ford Mechanic?

Most likely you said Porsche!

WHY?

Even though both know how to work on engines!

Porsche **is** their <u>area of expertise!</u>

The same holds true when it comes to *depression*:

Even though primary care doctors know medicine,

Depression is a psychiatrist's <u>**area of expertise**</u>!

Does that make sense?

When it comes to **Outpatient Treatment** here are some things you can do that will make sure you stay depressed!

Of course to get well you want to *do the opposite!*

To stay depressed:

- ✓ Don't even seek help in the **1st** place.
- ✓ Miss appointments.
- ✓ Don't call to cancel appointments.
- ✓ Don't communicate openly and honestly
- ✓ Don't reschedule another appointment
- ✓ **DROP OUT** of treatment
- ✓ Stay in treatment you don't think is working but don't talk to anyone about it.

Most important to getting well!

1. Make all appointments - **(Whether you feel like it or not!)**

2. Be **open & honest** in communications

3. If you must cancel an appointment, *reschedule right way.*

4. **Talk** about your idea to stop treatment.

5. Let your provider know if you feel like what you doing is **NOT** working for you.

6. Remember:
   Treatment can take some time.
   Feeling better won't happen overnight!

#5) Sobriety

When it comes to *not using* <u>any</u> drugs or alcohol

It is your decision to make.

I *will not* tell another person what *they* should do!

What I *will do* is

point out a couple of important facts!!

Oil & water **DO NOT** mix well together!

Likewise…….

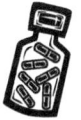

Antidepressant medication

&

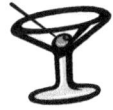

alcohol (or other drugs)

DO NOT mix well together!

If you read the warnings of the medication -

many pharmaceutical companies will tell you

not to drink while taking their medication.

If you are working with a prescriber to try and **get your symptoms stabilized** with medications, it is required that you abstain from

all alcohol until that happens.

If you find you are unable to stop using –

it might mean this is more of an issue for you than

'JUST RELAXING'

If you want **help** with an alcohol or drug problem,

there are many types of **help** available including:

Medications to help with cravings

Treatment programs

Self help organizations

Please talk with your treatment provider

#6) Structure

Just as with the other 3 other corner foundations- this will **make or break** your recovery.

One good way to think about structure is:

"What routines do you follow?"

Another good way to think about it is "What do you do with your time?"

For a lot of people, structure is created by **work, school, family obligations**.

But what happens when that changes or you don't have it to start with?

Or

Are you one of those people who has **too much** to do in too little time?

Structure is **critical** to recovery. It's really 2 steps:

1. Having a daily structure in place
2. Making sure it is 'balanced'

When it comes to **Structure** here are some things you can do that will make sure you stay depressed!

Of course to get well you want to *do the opposite!*

To stay depressed:

- ✓ Wake up when you want
- ✓ Don't have any plan or structure to your day.
- ✓ Have **too much free time** on your hands.
- ✓ Try to take on **too** many things in the day
- ✓ Stay in bed or in the bedroom all day.
- ✓ Watch TV 12 hours a day......

Most important to getting well!

1. Set the alarm and wake up at a consistent time (No longer than 1 extra hour on weekends!)

2. Have a **daily schedule** written out & follow it!

3. If you are not working, make sure to fill the daily plan with other activities – **volunteer!**

4. If a parent, create some 'me' time - even if it's just five minutes.

5. Limit the television you watch.

6. Get outside for 15 minutes.

7. Do not isolate yourself in one room.

8. Make sure you have the **other parts** of the **Wellness Blueprint ™** planned in your day.

9. Use a daily or weekly calendar

10. Work on household chores even if for only **5** minutes at a time!

Building the
Rest of the Foundation!

#7) Nutrition

There are 2 types of nutrients our bodies need that tend to get very affected by depression:

Food & Sleep

When it comes to *Food* –

Depression can take our eating behaviors in the opposite directions-

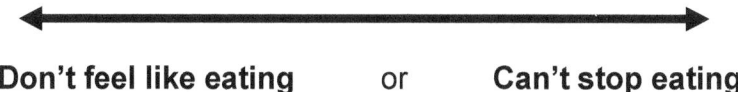

Don't feel like eating   or   **Can't stop eating**

Neither one of these will help us get better!

An important consideration is that some medications will increase people's cravings for sweets – usually leading to more junk food!!

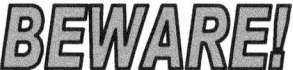

It's not just the medicine that puts the weight on;

it's *what we put in our mouths too!*

If you notice:

You're eating healthy, exercising, & still gaining weight *talk to your prescriber* about the issue.

** A good prescriber **should be** concerned with weight gain.

The other nutrient our bodies need is sleep!

When it comes to *Sleep* –

Depression can take our sleeping patterns in the opposite directions-

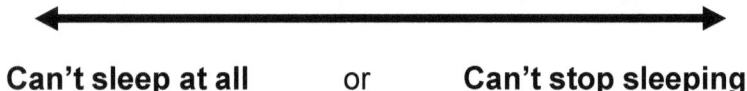

Can't sleep at all   or   **Can't stop sleeping**

The problem here is 'not sleeping' can have such an immediate impact on our emotional well being,

This can often be what leads people to self medicating with drugs or alcohol –

so they *can* get some sleep.

When it comes to **Nutrition** here are some things you can do that will make sure you stay depressed!

Of course to get well you want to *do the opposite!*

To stay depressed:

- ✓ Keep *self medicating* to go to sleep.

- ✓ Eat based on how you feel ---
  - If you're **hungry** – **eat**!
  - If you're **not hungry** – **don't eat**!

- ✓ Drink as much caffeine as you can!

- ✓ Eat ALL the JUNK FOOD you like.

- ✓ *Don't* talk to your prescriber about your sleep problems.

- ✓ Keep sleeping as <u>much as you feel like.</u>

- ✓ *Take long naps* day after not sleeping well!

Most important to getting well!

1. Talk to a health care provider about your sleep problems.

2. Manage your diet to **3** meals a day.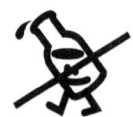

3. **Eat** a little bit – even if you're **not hungry**.

4. **Limit** the caffeine and junk food!

5. Stop self medicating for sleep.

6. *Do not* sleep during the day after a night you can't sleep.

7. Do not sleep longer than 8 – 10 hours; make yourself get out of bed.

8. If you wake up at night & cannot fall back asleep, go sit in another room until you feel tired.
   DO NOT: Smoke, clean house, or be active!

9. If your mind won't shut off, try *journaling* or *relaxation techniques*

#8) Exercise

Another good way to think about exercise is think

Activity!

Exercise doesn't have to be just going to a gym

or doing **aerobics**

or WEIGHTS

or Running

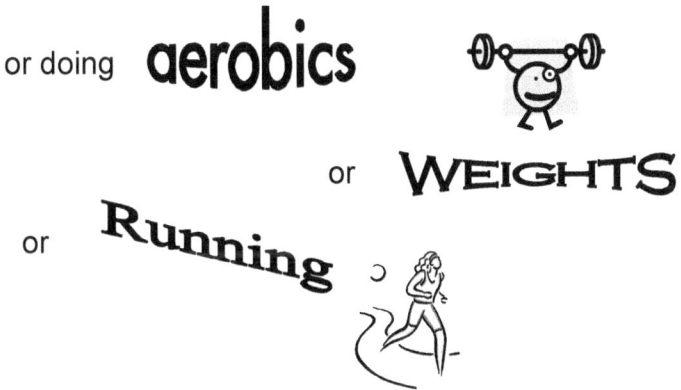

Here, it is about **increasing our level of activity!!**

There are plenty of ways to do this

without too much inconvenience!!

Now – don't get me wrong!   I am **not** saying:

"*Don't* go to the gym, do aerobics, or go running!"

If you *can* and *are* doing that – GREAT!

Keep it up!!!!

When it comes to **Exercise** here are some things you can do that will make sure you stay depressed!

Of course to get well you want to *do the opposite!*

To stay depressed:

- ✓ **Stop** exercise routines completely

- ✓ Park your car at the *closest spot possible*!

- ✓ Have someone else do your shopping & chores

- ✓ Stay a **couch or bed potato!**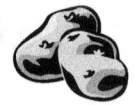

Most important to getting well!

1) When sitting in a chair watching TV, pick your feet up and down through the commercials – gradually build you're way up in time.

2) Do some extra housecleaning = ↑
   ACTIVITY!

3) Take the elevators up but the stairs
   D
     O
       W
         N

4) Walk to your mailbox a couple of times a day!

5) Take the dog for a walk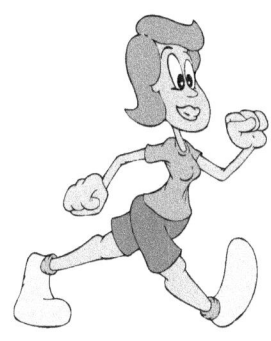

6) Park ⟶ f u r t h e r   a w a y!

7) Walk in-place during TV commercials!

#9) Support

This is such an important area.

It can have a significant impact on recovery –

Both **positive & negative**

One of the ways I help people understand the impact of not having support is the following:

> Parlez Vous Francaise?

Have you ever been around a group of people who were speaking in another language you didn't understand *at all*?

How did you *feel*? What were you *thinking*?

I had this experience on a trip to see my brother, who, thanks to the Navy, was stationed in Italy.

I felt VERY anxious!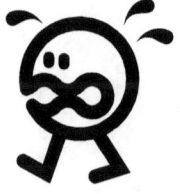

What would I do if I got lost or separated?

I also felt helpless, powerless and a little paranoid!

How would I be able to **ask for help**?

What were they saying about me?

The point is *people who experience depression* also **speak a different language**.

Not being around people who can speak & understand it can leave *you* feeling **alone, helpless, & powerless**.

Sometimes, family members are able to understand the language.

More times than not, they just are *not able* to but not for lack of wanting to!!

? After all, **?**

It's hard to speak a language if you don't know it?!

And it may take them a little time to learn it!!!

When it comes to **Support** here are some things you can do that will make sure you stay depressed!

Of course to get well you want to *do the opposite!*

To stay depressed:

- ✓ **Don't** have anyone around you who can **understand depression.**

- ✓ Stay connected to toxic people.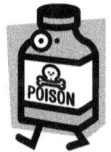

- ✓ Listen to people who tell you to "**snap out of it**" or to "**stop taking the medication**".

- ✓ Believe you are the only one having this problem.

- ✓ Have **NO SUPPORTS** at all!

Most important to getting well!

1) Let family and friends know when they say things that don't feel supportive.

2) If there is a group available at your outpatient treatment setting, ask to join in.

3) Join in online forums and groups.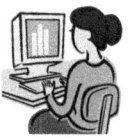

4) Get involved in:
   NAMI (National Alliance for Mentally Ill) or **DBSA**. (Depression Bipolar Support Alliance)

   See Additional Resources for contact information

5) If possible, have a *family session* with your outpatient provider.

6) Help **educate others** so they better understand about mental illness.

7) ✓ if your local hospital has any support groups you can get involved with.

#10) Socialization

The opposite of socialization is ISOLATION!

This is the key thing we need to address.

Isolation is to depression

what a gasoline is to a fire –

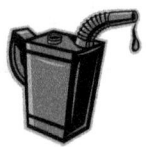 **an accelerant!**

Isolation has a way of *fueling* the depression,

making it even worse....

What makes it particularly challenging is the fact that

isolation

is also a symptom of depression.

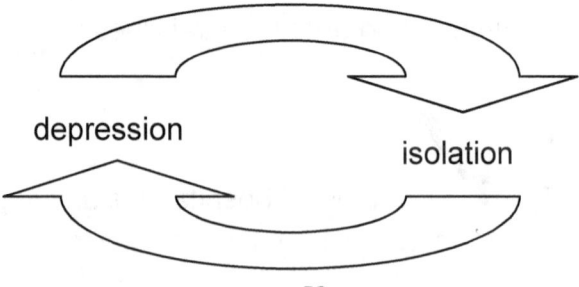

Now, I'm not saying we have to become a social butterfly!

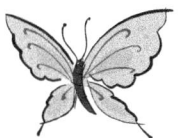

But we do have to take steps & actions to make sure we are not isolating.

When it comes to **Socialization** here are some things you can do that will make sure you stay depressed!

Of course to get well you want to *do the opposite!*

To stay depressed:

- ✓ Continue avoiding **family & friends**
- ✓ Keep yourself hidden away in your home.
- ✓ Turn off your phone.

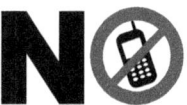

- ✓ Pull down all the shades.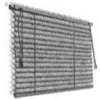

- ✓ Don't return phone messages or emails.

- ✓ **Avoid** the mailbox and computer.

- ✓ Stop going to social types of gathering

- ✓ Stay **isolated** in one room.

- ✓ **STOP!** going to religious services.

Most important to getting well!

1. Start spending **small amounts** of time outside the room you were isolated in.

2. Turn the phone back on and answer it!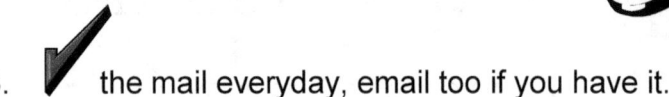

3. ✓ the mail everyday, email too if you have it.

4. Make a point to **reach out to** at least 1 person.

5. Send a letter, email, or card to someone.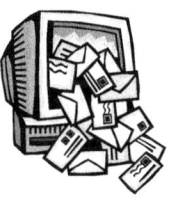

6. Join an online community!

7. **At least go** to a social function – leave early if you must.

8. Talk with someone from your religious organization

9. Call a helpline.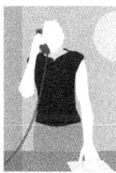

10. Go spend time in the library.

11. Say *hello* to at least one person a day!

12. **STOP ISOLATING!**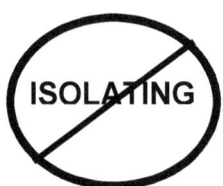

#11) Coping skills

I believe there are 2 types of coping skills:

"**Survival tools**"   &   "**LifeTools**".

Survival tools refer to the coping skills we tend to develop *out of the necessity* to deal with a problem or issue in our lives.

Early in my life **alcohol** was one of my **survival tools**. It was the way I found to cope with my father's death.

The problem with **Survival tools:** *they* tend to become a **problem** themselves!

What once may have helped us cope, can turn around and start to hurt us.

Which brings me to the **LifeTools**!

These are the **healthy** coping skills

we must develop to replace the old survival tools!

Fortunately, I was able to replace

my survival tool, alcohol, with a LifeTool, basketball.

How do you deal with stress, your emotions,

problems or issues going on in your life?

Unless *we are* managing

our stress, emotions, life problems & issues

they will be managing us!

Just as isolation **FUELS** the illness

So too does our **stress**, our **emotions** & **life issues**.

Healthy coping skills minimize their impact!

When it comes to **Coping Skills** here are some things you can do that will make sure you stay depressed!

Of course to get well you want to *do the opposite!*

To stay depressed:

- ✓ Hold everything inside

- ✓ Keep using your old "**Survival Tools**"!

- ✓ Continue to *BLAME* everyone else for your problems.

- ✓ When you get **stressed out** or angry - **eat, drink, and smoke more!**

- ✓ Refuse to see how the survival tools may be hurting you

- ✓ Avoid dealing with things

- ✓ **Don't change.**

Most important to getting well!

1. Take **100%** responsibility for your actions and emotions.

2. Be **open** to trying new ways of coping.

3. Instead of avoiding things – Deal with them!

4. Try talking or writing about how you feel.

5. Take a 👓 at what is working & what is not.

6. Replace old survival tools with new life tools.

7. Break **big** problems and issues down in to **small piles**.

8. Be willing to & do **ask for help.**

#12) Communication

If I could teach only one skill to people, this is it!

Let's face it –

it's nearly impossible to just get through a day

without **communicating!**

I believe the **QUALITY** of life is greatly influenced

by the **QUALITY** of our communication skills.

What I see as most important is

our ability to express our needs and emotions.

(No one can know what they are until we say them!)

There are **3** basic approaches in communication:

Aggressive

Assertive

Passive

Aggressive: My needs and wants are all that matters! It is my way or no way.

Passive: My needs and wants aren't important at all. I'll just keep them to myself

Assertive: My needs and wants are just as important as your needs and wants are.

WAIT!
I forgot the 4th one!!

PASSIVE-AGGRESSIVE

This can actually be the **MOST DAMAGING** to our relationships

Because….

people do not express their needs & wants in a very direct way….

leading us to feel they're **not being honest** with us.

Behaviors speak louder than words!

Examples:

1) Rather than tell the waitress the service was poor – I don't leave a tip!

2) When you ask what is wrong -   I say **"nothing"** but my tone of voice & body language tells you "*something*" is!

3) Instead of telling you I am angry, I slam doors & drawers, make a lot of noise, or purposely do things to annoy you!

or

4) I communicate by *what I don't say*! the silent treatment, showing up late, or not calling when I am suppose to!

The other way I like to get people to think about it....

It's like someone trying to sneak in to your home through the " BACK "

when you would rather they just come directly in the front door rather than trying to be **SNEAKY.**

Which one describes you best?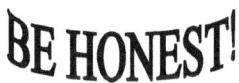

Another way I like to have people look at ways we can communicate......

Imagine we are both sitting at the table – sitting face to face across from one another.

How would you prefer to be 'served'?

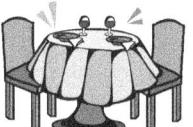

- I **shove** everything at you!

- I **set it** on the table in front of you so you can take what you want.

- I **don't put anything** on the table, leaving you with nothing at all.

or

- I set it in front of you then **take it away**, pretending it was never there in the first place!

Think about it...
How do you 'serve' other people?!

Do you need work on your **communication skills?**

When it comes to **Communication** here are some things you can do that will make sure you stay depressed!

Of course to get well you want to *do the opposite!*

To stay depressed:

- ✓ Believe that people *should know what you are thinking?*

- ✓ **Hold everything in** and don't speak up.

- ✓ Refuse to see the need to change.

- ✓ Keep **doing what** you've been doing.

- ✓ Believe that if he/she loved me, they wouldn't have to ask.

- ✓ Let your **emotions** come either roaring out or sneak out in subtle ways.

Most important to getting well!

1. Recognize that no one knows what you are thinking until you **tell them**.

2. Be willing to 'put things on the table', not shove them at someone.

3. Stop holding everything inside.

4. Don't let **emotions** build up!

5. Work on improving your communication skills.

6. If you can't express yourself verbally, try writing instead.

#13) Spirituality

The most important thing when it comes to spirituality: **It is up to us**, as individuals, **how we will define this**.

Years ago, I had a person offer a wonderful definition. It's the one I use to this very day!

"Spirituality is the way or ways in which we create an inner sense of peace."

For some people that is religious services.

For others it may be prayer, meditation, readings, or listening to recordings.

*** A special note – It is not medicine related peace!***

I once had a patient tell me that's what her Xanax did for her & they took it away!

Do you have any spiritual practices?
Did you have them & then STOP
as the depression got worse?

Maybe you feel like this area does not apply to you.

I can respect that.

You simply move on to the next part of the foundation.

Most important to getting well!

1. Listen to some music that may connect for you.

2. Do some reading, even if it is just a quote.

3. Make a point to do **some small step** everyday.

4. Try to attend services a shorter period of time.

5. Engage in conversations about your spirituality.

#14) Leisure

One of the things I've noticed is that when symptoms start to get worse, people's leisure interests/activities stop.

Leisure plays a very important role in wellness & recovery for several reasons:

1 It can often be what we use to create structure in our free time.

2 It helps feed so many of our values & needs.

3 It can act as a balancing force in our lives:
Example: Work and play
Us and them
Indoors and outside
Activity and inactivity

What are some of the things you **used to like to do**?

How did you **used to feel doing them**?

When it comes to **Leisure** here are some things you can do that will make sure you stay depressed!

Of course to get well you want to *do the opposite!*

To stay depressed:

- ✓ **Wait** to do things again until you 'feel' like it.

- ✓ Spend all your free time either in bed or watching TV

- ✓ When you're feeling bored – sleep.

- ✓ Stay indoors! Do not step outside at all!

- ✓ Remain **unwilling** to try new things

Most important to getting well!

1. **Start small!** *Every little thing counts!*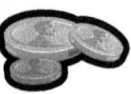

2. ***DO THEM! Even if you don't feel like it!***

3. Push yourself to start doing leisure activities again.

4. **Limit the amount** of time you sleep and watch TV

5. Step outside! Even if it's just for 2 minutes.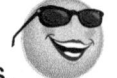

6. **Get active!** Do something requires you move.

7. Don't expect to pick up where you left off.

8. Be p a t i e n t with yourself!

9. **Dig out** the interests that got buried in the depression!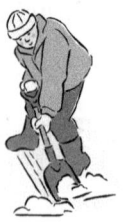

#15) Acceptance

I may be able to convince you to try &
follow the Wellness Blueprint™ for a short while -

yet

if you are going to continue this wellness - recovery
work for any longer period of time….

(for me it's *the rest of my life* &
I hope the same for you!)

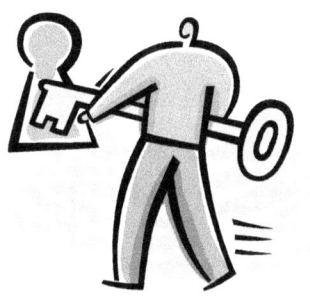

the key is

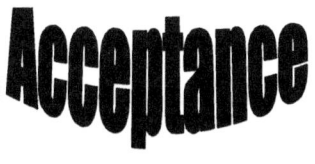

Let's be clear…'acceptance' does not mean **'<u>like</u>'**!

I haven't meant anyone who **LIKES** being depressed!!

What acceptance means is

recognizing the depression is part of our lives

&

we need to **learn how to live with it**.

My experiences have taught me we all don't reach this place of acceptance the same way!

For some people, it might be easier than for others.

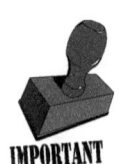

We should not judge either ourselves or anybody else.

The important question I have to ask you is this:

Is what you are doing in your life right now working?

Be honest!!

If it **is** – great!   Don't change a thing!

If it **isn't** – how about *making some changes!*

When it comes to **Acceptance** here are some things you can do that will make sure you stay depressed!

Of course to get well you want to *do the opposite!*

To stay depressed:

- ✓ Keep asking yourself "***Why me?***"

- ✓ Continue to play the *'blame game'*

- ✓ Hold on to the attitude **'it's not fair'**

- ✓ See things aren't working but <u>don't change.</u>

- ✓ **Ignore** all the warning signs

- ✓ Believe you are *the only one* with this problem.

Most important to getting well!

1. **Stop** asking yourself 'why me'

2. Understand this is an *illness* **NOT WEAKNESS**

3. Recognize how *blaming* will keep you stuck.

4. Remember:
   It's not what happens to us but what we *do* about it!

5. Be *open & willing* to change what is not working.

6. ***Get involved*** with a support group – you aren't the only one.

7. Continue to work towards acceptance.

8. Realize you are in some famous company! Mental illness ***does not*** discriminate!

#16) Self Esteem

Last but not least – self esteem!

The simple definition I use for self esteem
"How we *feel about ourselves*"

Something I've noticed with self esteem & depression:
There are 2 groups people seem to fit in to.

In the first group are the people
who had good self esteem until they got depressed.

It went 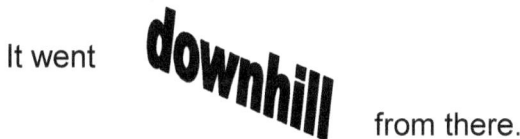 from there.

The second group of people are different.

Self esteem didn't go down when they got depressed
because they didn't have very much to begin with.

The bad news here is it will take a *little more work*.

I like to get people thinking of building self esteem as being like growing flowers..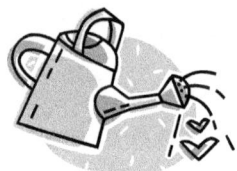

It all starts with planting 'seeds'!

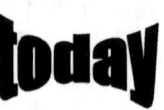

From there it requires 'care and feeding' in order to grow!

Some people were fortunate -
They had seeds planted when they were young.

Others were *not so fortunate*...

We can't go back and change the past...

we can only take care of **today**

It is **never too late** to start planting!

When it comes to **Self Esteem** here are some things you can do that will make sure you stay depressed!

Of course to get well you want to *do the opposite!*

To stay depressed:

- ✓ Continue to **see ourselves as a victim** of a bad childhood (if it applies).

- ✓ Engage in **negative** and critical self talk.

- ✓ Let how other people see you, be how you see yourself.

- ✓ Blame other people for the way you feel.

- ✓ Remain the biggest bully to yourself.

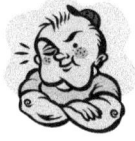

- ✓ Stay in a toxic and unhealthy relationship.

- ✓ Allow people to be abusive to you.

- ✓ Let others make decisions **FOR YOU**.

- ✓ Base your self esteem on outside things... like a job, income, role, possessions, success.

Most important to getting well!

1. Do some type of **self care** activity every day.

2. Take complete responsibility for your feelings.

3. Stay **focused** on **today** & catch yourself when you start to think of the past.

4. Replace ▬ and critical self talk with ✚ and supportive self talk.

5. Start to make your own decisions.

6. Recognize what's happened in the past **does not** make you a victim today.

7. Stay away from toxic people.

8. Set limits and say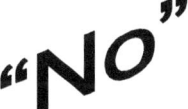

9. Do not allow your illness to define WHO you are!

R
e
m
e
m
b
e
r

1. Plant the seeds!

2. Water daily!

#17) Putting It All Together!

So there you have it!

The Wellness Blueprint ™ laid out for you to follow.

When it comes to putting these things in place it all comes down to "**Baby Steps**"!

By taking '**small actions**' every day we are building that foundation a little bit at a time!

Brick by brick!

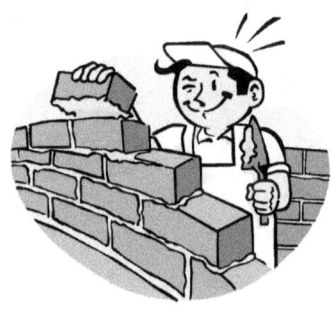

I guarantee

that if you follow the blueprint…

You will feel much better!

After all,

it *is* what has helped keep me well all these years!

A BONUS GIFT!

We have a special bonus for you!

Go to:

www.TheWellnessBlueprint.com/MeasuringTape

Put your name and email in the box

Click "Send Me My Measuring Tape Carol!"

Once you have confirmed it is okay to add you to our email server, we will send you an email containing **an assessment you can use to measure the strength of your wellness foundation & areas to focus on!**

Be on the lookout -

It will come from Well YOUniversity!

You can always reach us at:

Mail@TheWellnessBlueprint.com

Additional Resources

1. **NAMI**   www.nami.org

   NAMI is the National Alliance on Mental Illness, the nation's largest grassroots organization for people with mental illness and their families. Founded in 1979, NAMI has affiliates in every state and in more than 1,100 local communities across the country. NAMI is dedicated to the eradication of mental illnesses and to the improvement of the quality of life for persons of all ages who are affected by mental illnesses.

2. **DBSA**   www.dbsalliance.org

   The Depression and Bipolar Support Alliance is the leading patient-directed national organization focusing on the most prevalent mental illnesses. The organization fosters an environment of understanding about he impact and management of these life-threatening illnesses by providing up-to-date, scientifically-based tools and information written in language the general pubic can understand. DBSA supports research to promote more timely diagnosis, develop more effective and tolerable treatments and discover a cure. The organization works to ensure that people living with mood disorders are treated equitably. DBSA was founded in 1985.

3. **MHA**   www.nmha.org

   Mental Health America (formerly known as the National Mental Health Association) is the country's leading nonprofit dedicated to helping ALL people live mentally healthier lives. With our more than 320 affiliates nationwide, we represent a growing movement of Americans who promote mental wellness for the health and well-being of the nation – everyday and in times of crisis.

4. **BP Hope Magazine**   www.BPHope.com

   BP Magazine offers bipolar disorder information, support, and bipolar resources for patients, family, and friends in each issue.

5. **Esperanza**   www.hopetocope.com

   From the publisher's of BP Magazine, a unique magazine for those living with depression and anxiety, seeking hope, understanding and support. Each issue will focus on the unique needs and wants of an estimated 40 million Americans, and so many others throughout the world, living with anxiety and depression.

6. **NIMH**   www.nimh.nih.gov

   The National Institute of Mental Health is the largest scientific organization in the world dedicated to research focused on understanding, treatment, and prevention of mental disorders and the promotion of mental health.

About Well YOUniversity, LLC

We are a company dedicated to
restoring hope, health, & happiness
to those struggling with chronic health conditions.

Our mission is to improve an individual's quality of life by helping them develop the knowledge, skills, & supports needed to improve maximize their health.

We accomplish this by offering products and services
that inspire & empower our clients
in achieving lifelong wellness.

Please visit us at www.WellYOUniversity.com

Share Your Success Story

The are so many people out there, struggling along.
You can help them by
sharing your success using the Wellness Blueprint!

Go to
www.TheWellnessBlueprint.com/success
and let us all know you're taking back
CONTROL OF YOUR LIFE!

www.ingramcontent.com/pod-product-compliance
Lightning Source LLC
LaVergne TN
LVHW051849080426
835512LV00018B/3151